You've counted calories.

You've gorged yourself on protein, then on carbohydrates.

You've dieted on grapefruit, chocolate and bananas.

You've run around the block for hours.

You've attended weekly meetings.

You've wasted money on expensive exercise machines.

You've drunk gallons of shakes.

You've gulped a thousand pills.

You've eaten a thousand meal replacement bars.

You've kept a weight loss journal or blog.

You've bought tiny plates to make your food portions look big.

You've spent thousands of dollars on special foods.

You've stapled your ears.

But you're still overweight.

Maybe you lost some pounds, but regained that fat, and more.

Now it's time to stop working so hard to lose weight and try it the easy way.

Relax and Lose Weight

It's the only way.

No jogging for miles.

No jumping around to a cardio DVD.

No tedious diets.

No special foods to buy.

No calories to count.

No fighting your cravings.

Stop stressing out about your weight. Relax and let your thin self loose.

Relax to Lose Weight

How to Shed Pounds Without Starvation Dieting, Gimmicks or Dangerous Diet Pills, Using the Power of Sensible Foods, Water, Oxygen and Self-Image Psychology

Melissa Martin

ISBN: 1451593295

EAN-13: 9781451593297

LEGAL NOTICE

Disclaimer

I am not a doctor, a nurse, a chiropractor, or even a hospital janitor.

I'm not a personal trainer or nutritionist.

I've never won any bodybuilding or beauty contests. I have no fancy degrees or certifications.

I am a researcher, journalist and writer with a wide range of knowledge based on what's worked for me, and what I've learned from a variety of fields.

This program includes elements of nutritional research, exercise research, self-image psychology, neuro-linguistic programming, and physiological research.

I've "borrowed" from the best to provide you with the most comprehensive—and yet easiest—weight loss program on the market.

To the best of my knowledge, everything in this program is factual and effective.

However, I make no claim of diagnosing or curing any medical conditions.

Everybody should consult with their physician before making any changes to their diet or before beginning any kind of exercise program.

This goes double if you are now taking any medication. You

should be monitored by a qualified medical professional.

This goes triple if you're already suffering from a weight related medical condition such as arthritis, diabetes, heart disease, or high blood pressure.

Many overweight people have mental and emotional issues that affect their weight. This book does not profess to replace a psychologist, psychiatrist or counselor. If you need a mental health professional, get help immediately.

I don't know you personally. Nothing in this book is or should be construed as personal medical advice.

This book is written as a source of information to educate the reader. Neither the author nor the publisher shall be liable or responsible for any adverse effects arising from the use or application of any of the information contained herein, nor do they guarantee that everyone will lose weight with these techniques, and are not responsible if they do not.

This book is written as a source of information to educate the reader. It is not intended to replace professional medical advice.

The author has no financial ties to any of the products or services cited.

The author and publisher shall not be liable or responsible for any adverse effects arising from the use or application of any of the information herein. Nor do they guarantee that everyone will benefit or lose weight with this advice.

Continuing to read this book implies acceptance of these terms.

Table of Contents

Introduction

Maybe so many Americans (and millions of other people around the world) are obese because losing weight has been made to seem like such hard work.

Going to meetings, counting calories, running until we drop, counting fat grams, keeping a journal (which often includes writing down every single bite you took during the day), buying (and using) expensive exercise machines...whew!

I don't know about you, but I need to eat a lot of calories just to keep up with the typical weight loss program.

We're stressed out enough by the rest of our lives. Heck, we're stressed out by being overweight. Who wants to add more items to their "To Do List?"

I don't want to add stress to your life. I don't want you to count calories. I don't want you to go to meetings. I don't want you to run long, boring hours as "cardio." I don't want to control every bite of what you eat. I don't want you to write a food blog or journal. I don't want you to waste money on diet pills. If you like certain protein bars or shakes and they're convenient to eat on the run, that's fine, but they're not required. I don't want you to pay for a gym membership or an exercise machine.

Most of what I'll ask you to do consists of—are you ready for this?—sitting down and relaxing.

Obesity is a serious problem.

Why Do You Want to Lose Weight

According to experts in the field, people want to lose weight for many reasons. But boiled down, there're only two:

1. You want to look better.

2. You fear current or future health problems caused by carrying excess pounds.

I wrote this book to help you look and feel better—the simple and easy way.

Weight loss should be simple and easy—or it won't last.

That's why too many people see their weight bounce up and down like yo-yos—they get so exhausted from their weight loss programs they have to stop and rest, and so the weight soon returns.

Look at it this way...

If your goal is just immediate weight loss, you can achieve that simply by spending the next entire twenty-four hours fasting (don't even drink any water) and exercising (walk as far as you can, stop and rest, continue walking).

You'll lose weight all right, but will you keep it off? Probably not. The next day, you'll sleep all morning and then eat three times as much food as normal.

The Seed of This Book

Late last year I read a dieting book that gave a weight loss "tip" that enraged me.

Because all physical activity burns up calories, this book advised readers to be constantly moving some part of their body. That means tapping their feet or twitching their fingers. Work, church, movie theaters or any other place where you can't accomplish any major physical movement are perfect for this.

The author's rationale is that all such movement burns calories. Yes, of course tapping your finger all day doesn't use up a lot of calories—but the calories it does burn are calories you no longer need to lose.

And over time, those calories can add up to a significant amount of weight that's no longer on your body.

So why did that advice outrage me?

Maybe it's because I have a tendency to be nervous. Continuously tapping your finger is not a healthy activity.

Besides, if you're in a public place you may be a stress "spreader." I know many times at work and in other places, I've been stressed out by people's nervous habits, including nonstop shifting around in their chairs and tapping their fingers (especially drumming their fingernails).

What's even worse is that acting nervous not only bugs the people around you, but our own feelings tend to correspond to our physical states. So when we act nervous, we FEEL nervous.

If you're always jittery, people won't notice and admire you for losing weight—they'll be too busy trying to move away from you because you make them feel nervous.

What's the point of losing weight if you're always acting like a cokehead who hasn't snorted a line in two weeks?

And how can you have perfect health when you're all stressed out?

You can't.

Sometimes what seems like a good idea doesn't work in real life.

Weight Loss is About a Lot More Than Food and Blood Sugar Levels

Here's another example that affected my thinking, eventually leading to this book.

In my opinion, the best eating plan to lose weight and improve your health is the Zone Diet by Dr. Barry Sears.

I've read all his books. I've been on it as much as practically possible. And I have lost a lot of weight—38 pounds in the past seven months.

So it works. I absolutely believe it's the healthiest way for everybody to eat. But one thing Dr. Sears says in his books irritates me.

Perhaps it's because of his scientific training.

According to research, he writes, we feel "hungry" when our blood sugar levels fall below a certain amount.

The Zone Diet advises you to eat what you need and no more, spreading your meals throughout the day. According to Dr. Sears, this will prevent your blood sugar levels from falling far enough to make you feel hungry from one meal to the next.

According to Dr. Sears, the Zone Diet keep your blood sugar over "hunger signal" levels. Therefore, you don't feel hungry between meals. So you aren't tempted to eat too much.

Yeah, right.

I knew it was B.S. the first time I read it. And my own experiences with the Zone Diet reinforces that opinion.

I keep to the Zone as much as I can—enough to lose 38 pounds in 7 months—but I'm perfectly capable of feeling hunger almost right after eating a full meal for men (according to the Zone plan), even though I'm a woman.

I used to deliver pizzas. Sometimes I'd eat a (Zone) Balance Bar while on a delivery, then return to the store and still have room to stuff my face with several slices of a "mistake" pizza.

I've never tickled my throat to induce vomiting so I could stuff even more food down my mouth, as ancient Romans reputedly did. However, I have many times felt totally full—even stuffed—after one plate, then gone back to the line for a second plate full of food.

I'm willing to bet you've done that too.

The Zone Diet worked for me, but not because every Zone meal and snack made me feel "just" satisfied when I really wanted to feel stuffed to the gills.

It worked because I combined it with meditation and other

techniques I've learned over the years.

That brings home the point an effective diet is not just about the food you eat, or even how much food you eat.

Those things are important, but what's going on inside your head has the most effect on your diet's ultimate, long-term success or failure.

And yet your mind is blocked because you've been brainwashed into thinking losing weight is hard work.

Wouldn't it be great, I thought, if somebody could write a book about losing weight the EASY way?

So I did.

You're welcome.

Chapter 1

Why Lose Weight

Weight loss experts know the two major reasons people want to lose weight are:

1. To improve appearance

2. To improve health

I suspect most people have both these motivations, but one or the other predominates.

Some people argue we should ignore #1 because it's politically incorrect. We should see the value in people based on who they are on the inside—on their character and personality.

I can't really say those people are wrong, because this area is subjective.

For the record, I love, honor, cherish the inner beauty and appreciate the intelligence and character of many people... old and young, men and women, of all races, weak and strong, conventionally beautiful and conventionally ugly, thin and fat— but that doesn't mean I want to have sex with all or any of them.

Yes, it's true many people are in a gray area. They're not physically attractive at first glance, but when you get to know and like them the idea of sex with them becomes more comfortable, even attractive.

So, within limits, I do agree #1 should not be important.

But since when did most people do what they *should* do?

We're Affected by Physical Appearances, Probably More Than We Admit

Let's face it, when I'm walking around a shopping center or on the beach it's not a guy's inner personality that catches my eye and makes my heart thump and my vagina moisten—it's his broad shoulders, muscular chest and six pack abs.

I absolutely agree beauty is subjective and many men vary in their own sexual desires more than the mainstream media would have us believe. Not all men want a perfect 36-24-36 Barbie doll. Not even most.

Some men do prefer a three hundred pound woman.

But if your particular partner/husband/boyfriend prefers a hundred thirty pound woman and you're three hundred pounds, you've got a situation to deal with.

And if you don't have a partner/husband/boyfriend and you want one, you're much more likely to attract favorable male attention if you weigh one hundred thirty pounds than if you weigh three hundred.

It's a simple matter of odds. Because fewer men want three hundred pounds, they're harder to find.

Yes, the Internet has made this process a lot easier than it used to be. However, it's also true you're looking for men who have other favorable qualities besides lusting after your flesh. The more of those you can meet and date, the more likely you are to find not only one who lusts for you, but one you lust for in return.

There are also many studies verifying in our "shallow" society good looking people (body weight is not all of this, but part of it) get promoted more often, make more money and are more liked and trusted.

I Agree Health Is Most Important

These days, however, many women are not focused on what other people (men or women) think of them—they're concerned about themselves, including health.

So I have no problem with women making the politically correct choice to not lose weight to adhere to the body profile standards of the mainstream media and most men.

However, I must part company with the line of political correctness which claims body size is simply an individual choice and heavy people would all be fine of society would just stop "oppressing" them by telling them they should lose weight.

I'm totally against all forms of discrimination.

However, obese people aren't nearly as oppressed by society as they are by the extra fat cells in their bodies.

The medical evidence is clear, political correctness notwithstanding. Excess weight is a health risk.

So Reason #2 for losing weight is the most important, at least in my opinion. After all, you won't care how you look to people when you're dead.

The negative health effects of excess weight are many.

Increased risk of coronary heart disease, sleep apnea, diabetes, fatty liver disease, gout, arthritis, stroke, higher blood pressure, some cancers, gallstones, injuries from falling and more.

Pregnant obese women are more than twice as likely to suffer from blood clots in the lungs, which can be fatal.

Obese people are at greater risk during surgery because even minor procedures are more difficult.

Recently I read a fascinating book HOW NOT TO DIE by Dr. Jan Garavaglia, M.D., a long time medical examiner. She's performed thousands of autopsies.

She tells how the obese corpses she examines all have enlarged hearts, yellow-tinged granules of cholesterol in their coronary arteries and sacs of diverticulosis in their colons.

Obesity is Either a Cause of, Or Another Medical Condition Associated with Insulin Resistance

Current medical research is showing many conditions we think of as separate diseases are really related manifestations of insulin resistance caused by eating too many carbohydrates and keeping the body in a state of permanent inflammation.

I have a friend who's worked a long time for a welfare agency taking disability applications. She tells me when an obese woman sit down at her desk she could write half the application by rote: arthritis, high blood pressure, diabetes and, often heart problems and/or cancer.

She says she connected the dots between these conditions long before medical science started talking about Metabolic Syndrome or Syndrome X.

Most people who begin diet programs such as Weight Watchers and Jenny Craig, buy diet books, take diet pills and sign up for weight loss programs are women.

Therefore, most experts conclude it's mainly women who want to lose weight.

I believe this is only a partial truth.

Men Want to Lose Weight Too But They Call it "Building Muscle"

I suspect many men also want to look better and improve their health but they're just less likely to seek help (just as women go to the doctor a lot more than men).

After all, many men buy exercise programs promising them six pack abs. What are six pack abs but ordinary stomach muscles currently hiding behind a beer belly? The trainers selling these products understand men must lose a lot of fat to have the muscular body they desire.

Most men want to appear sexually attractive.

Most men want to live longer and in better physical condition.

They are more likely to take their health for granted and neglect their appearance than women, but may also be motivated to improve their appearance by a divorce or to improve their health by a diagnosis of high blood pressure.

They would be embarrassed to go to Jenny Craig, but men run, swim, cycle, lift weights, and go to gyms. They don't spend all that effort for nothing. They'll explain it's about health, fitness and building muscles—but that's just another way of saying "look sexier and have better health." So to me it's just another side of the same coin.

If you're a man, welcome!

This book is for you too.

The good news is everybody's health improves as soon as you start eating in a more healthy fashion.

You'll start looking better.

You'll start feeling better.

You'll reduce your risk of coronary heart disease, diabetes, arthritis and high blood pressure.

(NOTE: as mentioned in the Disclaimer, if you already have any of these conditions, check with your doctor before changing your diet.)

You'll have more energy.

You'll accomplish more, smile more, enjoy being with people more and enjoy life.

But it's up to you.

Chapter Two

You must Take Responsibility for Your Self

I have to confess something.

Although the theme of this book is losing weight the easy way, this chapter is not easy to act on.

It can be damned hard.

A lot harder than counting calories, writing a daily food blog or even running ten miles.

The good news is, it's the first and last truly difficult chore I'll demand you carry out.

Take the easy way out here, and nothing else you do will count, because it won't last.

You won't do what I advise. You'll probably just finish reading this, say "Good stuff," and throw the book down.

That's not what I want. That's not why I'm working so hard to finish writing this when I'd really rather watch a good movie.

You Must Assume Self-Responsibility

For your weight.

For your relationship with food.

For your relationship with your own body.

For everything that happens in your life.

It's YOUR life, not mine.

If you remain overweight, it's on your shoulders, not mine.

I feel for you. I want you to lose that excess fat. I really do, or I'd be watching a movie.

It's my responsibility to finish this book and make it as good as I can.

But it's your job to apply it to your own life.

See, lots of overweight people blame food (I had to finish all the food on my plate), or their upbringing (if I didn't eat everything on my plate, my mother thought I didn't love her), or their co-workers (Jenny would be insulted if I didn't eat any of the doughnuts she brought in), society (I have to eat fast food because I'm so busy), their spouse (if only he wouldn't irritate so much I wouldn't have to eat a bowl of chocolate fudge ice cream just to calm down), TV (I saw a pizza commercial so I had to call Domino's), the government (they should outlaw fatty foods so I can stop eating them), past attempts to lose weight (I regained the pounds when I stopped taking the pills) or fast food places (I had to order the supersized fries because they were a better bargain for the money).

The truth is, food doesn't force itself down your throat.

And nobody forces the food down your throat either. Not the farmers, the food companies or even your mother.

Marketing Works Hard to Influence You, but It Doesn't Control You

It's certainly true the food industry is widespread and controls a massive marketing machine that does everything in its power to convince you to eat more, and more often. And our emotional attachments to friends and family are intertwined with our emotional bonds to food.

That makes your job harder, but no less important.

When all's said and done, when you have trouble standing up from your easy chair nobody else can lift you up—just you.

So, resolve right here, right now—the future is going to be different from the past.

Right here, right now—take responsibility for yourself.

Acknowledge the Truth, Then Move Forward

Acknowledge this—you're overweight. You use food for emotional needs (entertainment, relaxation, comfort and stress reduction) instead of for the physical needs it is designed for. You haven't exercised enough. You've tried other weight loss programs but gained the weight back.

Whatever the unpleasant facts of your life are, acknowledge them—AND LOVE YOURSELF DESPITE ALL THESE PAST

MISTAKES!

I can't stress that enough. The object here is NOT to "blame yourself."

You've made mistakes. So what? I could write a thousand books about all the mistakes I've made.

Acknowledge your mistakes, learn from them and resolve to do better from this moment onward.

Because you do want a terrific, healthy slim future for yourself.

Because you do want to feel comfortable inside your body.

Because you want to reduce or prevent physical health problems caused by excess weight.

Because you want your family and friends to love you for your terrific, caring personality.

Because you friends and family love you and want the best for you, and so want you to feel good (even if they don't always seem so supportive).

Because when you have more physical energy you can have more fun and express more emotional love and happiness.

BECAUSE YOU DO LOVE YOURSELF.

That's the bottom line. You're a worthwhile person who deserves the best out of life. You've made mistakes—as everybody has—and you can learn from them.

If people couldn't learn from mistakes, we'd still be living in caves, or extinct.

Understanding your life is your life to take control of—and doing so!—is the hardest part.

Of life as well as losing weight.

Once that's out of the way, the rest is just a matter of details.

Let's get started.

We'll start with establishing a connection between stress and obesity.

The villain's name is cortisol.

Chapter Three

Cortisol, The Stress Hormone That Directly Connects Weight Loss to Relaxation

If you listened to the radio half as much as I have (I used to deliver pizzas), a few years ago you heard dozens of commercials for a weight loss product that promised to help us lose weight by reducing our levels of cortisol.

Cortisol is commonly known as the "stress hormone." That's because it's part of your body's natural response to stress.

Remember our bodies evolved hundreds of thousands of years ago, when life was more basic.

In those days, stress was not a mean boss who yelled at you. Stress was a giant bear rushing to kill you. Stress was seeing a crocodile headed toward your toddler. Stress was a dawn attack by a war party from the tribe next door.

Stress was an immediate, life or death situation.

Stress demanded an instant surge of energy, strength and speed. Heart beat goes up. Blood rushes to your muscles. You breath faster.

It's often called the "flight or fight" mechanism.

To help produce it, our adrenal glands secrete more cortisol. Cortisol raises our blood pressure, increases blood sugar and lowers our immune systems.

In short, cortisol helps your body respond to stress. It's relatively short-acting. Once the stress is over, we recover and go back to "normal."

In Today's World We Often Cannot Fight or Run Away

That's the problem in modern society.

Our primitive ancestors either survived danger or they didn't. And they probably didn't face enemies every day. Once they escaped (if they did), they returned to hunting, gathering and lying out in the sun.

Yet our mean boss is staring at us forty hours a week. We have to commute to work five days a week. We watch and hear the news 24/7 about thousands of people dying in floods, fires and earthquakes.

Cave people probably didn't worry much about the future—they didn't have IRAs, Social Security or Medicare. When they had plenty of food in their bellies, they could lie around in the sun.

Even when we're not experiencing direct stress, we're busy anticipating unpleasant future events.

Our bodies aren't designed for that. And cortisol is one reason why.

Too Much Cortisol Makes You Gain Weight

Chronically elevated levels of cortisol adversely affect your health in a number of ways, including reducing the strength of your immune system, making you prone to catch more diseases, and reducing your memory.

However, extra cortisol also makes you fat. Studies have shown injecting both animals and people with cortisol increases your appetite, makes you crave sugar and gain weight.

Ever gone home from a bad day at work and stuffed yourself with cake icing straight out of the can? I have.

There are a number of reasons for that.

1. Cortisol increases the amount of insulin in your blood.

Insulin is the hormone that tells your body to store calories as fat.

Therefore, excess levels of cortisol increases insulin resistance, making your body even more prone to store every bite of food you eat as fat cells.

2. Abdominal fat has four times as many cortisol receptors as the fat under your skin. Excess cortisol encourages the body to move fat from under your skin to deep inside your abdomen—and abdominal fat is harder to lose and more dangerous to your health.

3. Cortisol binds to receptors in the hypothalumus of your brain that stimulates you to eat food higher in sugar and fat.

4. Cortisol increases another substance that increases your

appetite: CRH (corticotrophin releasing hormone).

5. Cortisol decreases levels of leptin, and that increases your appetite.

So we've established that excess cortisol is bad for your health and especially your weight loss goals.

Now, what can you do about it?

Relaxing and Lowering Stress Reduces Cortisol

In part, this entire book is the answer to this question.

But first let's stick to cortisol, and you'll soon see why I say, "Relax to lose weight."

Studies have shown, besides chronic stress and anxiety, cortisol is raised to excess levels by caffeine, prolonged physical exercise, severe trauma and sleep deprivation.

Studies have also shown cortisol is reduced by laughing, getting a massage, meditating and listening to relaxing music.

Stress also encourages your body to gain weight, no matter what or how much you eat, by releasing a hormone called neuropeptide Y. That causes a buildup of abdominal fat.

I also suggest sitting back and watching a great horror/suspense/thriller/mystery movie.

Won't that stress you out? Yes—for a short time. But you always know it's just a movie. And in the end there's release and relaxation. That's why good suspense or horror thrillers have been popular movies since THE CABINET OF DR. CALIGARI.

It's a form of controlled stress, and we seem to have a large appetite for it. We loved to be scared, so long as we know the bogeyman is really wearing a fake mask and the blood of his victims is fake.

So, we've established scientifically stressing out about your excess weight is NOT the way to lose it.

Is it what we eat?

Chapter Four

What Diet To Go On

Now that we've linked stress to obesity, let's address the most obvious part of weight loss—what we eat.

Should you go on any particular diet?

I'm not telling you that. I can't. I'm not a doctor or weight loss researcher.

Here's my philosophy about it. You're free to think what you like.

As I mentioned in the introduction, I personally follow the Zone diet and have had great success with it. I believe it would work 99% of the time if I just stayed on it 100%, which I don't.

It makes the most sense to me, but I admit I'm not a medical expert.

I've read studies show people have lost weight on all the popular diets so long as they stay on them, and that makes sense too.

Many popular diets are variations of each other.

As Dr. Barry Sears writes in one of his books, there are basically only three—

1. Low fat and protein, high carbohydrate: Pritikin, Dean Ornish

2. Low carbohydrate, high fat and protein: Atkins

3. Moderate amounts of carbohydrates, fat and protein: Zone and South Beach

The Old-Fashioned, Common Sense Weight Loss Secret

I'm old enough to remember it used to be simple "common sense" fat people ate too many fat, sweet and starchy foods.

In those days, people who wanted to lose weight knew they had to stop eating candy, cakes, bread, rice, fried foods, spaghetti, barbecued ribs and potatoes—everything fatty, sweet or starchy.

Thanks to Nathan Pritikin and the United States Department of Agriculture, our biggest health enemy became "cholesterol"—and people cut down on meat and eggs, substituting huge amounts of grain-based meals for the now perceived as dangerous protein foods.

I'm not so sure Pritikin wanted people to eat lots of pasta. I've read Pritikin, and as I recall his ideal meal was a lot of vegetables "seasoned" with a small amount of meat.

(Sounds suspiciously like an ideal "Zone" meal to me. Could be Nathan Pritikin and Dr. Barry Sears are not as far apart as commonly believed?)

Dump the Pasta

But many people felt encouraged to eat lots more spaghetti in place of protein. After all, it didn't have any cholesterol in it. Suddenly, starchy foods were our friends.

Besides, who wanted to eat a plate of vegetables for dinner? Nobody.

I remember when "everybody" knew poor people were often overweight because they could afford to eat only macaroni and cheese, without the cheese.

A few decades later it is fashionable to eat macaroni as long as it is called by a fancier name. Hey, it makes you feel good. Once digested, starchy foods (only it's more fashionable to say, "high glycemic load" or highly dense carbohydrates) turn into sugar.

That sugar raises the blood sugar levels of your blood, which is dangerous. So your pancreas secretes lots of insulin. This hormone quickly drops your blood sugar levels, but signals your cells to store fat instead of burning it.

Not to mention chronically excessive levels of insulin cause insulin resistance which is the basis for many modern health problems.

Some pasta meals are worse for you than sugar. You'd never eat as much sugar in the form of candy bars as you do when you eat a plate full of spaghetti. (Well, maybe you did, but you won't any more...)

Rice is the same story. It's a food staple in Asia because it's filling and because peasants can't often eat chicken, beef, eggs or fish.

In America, it's fashionable. We think of Asian peasants as thin, so we forget rice has a high glycemic index.

Maybe we could still be thin as Asian peasants if we worked half as hard as they do, but we don't. (And upper class Asians who eat lots of rice without performing heavy stoop labor also get overweight.)

So, for what it's worth, my advice is simply to go back to the basics.

You Know the Foods You Shouldn't Eat - So Stop Eating Them

Avoid sweet, fatty, fried, starchy—all other foods you KNOW are not healthy.

Eat lean meats, fish, dairy products, vegetables and fruit.

Eat enough to feel full, but not stuffed.

Eat when you're really hungry or close to it, but not before.

Eat breakfast. (Many studies have shown this is important for losing weight and keeping it off.)

Don't eat after dinner/supper. If you have to stay up very late (as a pizza driver, I used to work until 3:00 AM on weekend nights), eat small, sensible snacks.

If you're busy and you've found some kind of weight loss shake or bar you find helps you, eat a sensible amount of them. I admit when I'm on the go I eat a lot of Zone diet Balance bars.

However, I must add that ONLY the original Balance line of bars available in stores such as Wal-Mart and online on sites such as Amazon and the bars available directly from Dr. Sears (see his website) are exactly Zone-balanced (40% carbohydrate, 30% protein, 30% fat). The others—even the ones calling themselves

Zone "Perfect"—are not. I've analyzed their labels.

If the bar meets Zone guidelines, the label will say it's 40/30/30 nutrition. If the label doesn't say that, it's not precisely a Zone bar. Which means it probably contains too many carbohydrates.

If you want to get more complicated, be my guest.

What about drinking instead of eating?

Alcohol is empty calories, the last thing you need—not to mention it lowers your inhibitions which encourages you to eat too much.

Coffee and tea contain caffeine, which raises cortisol the stress hormone. Bad!

Soda, "energy" drinks, fruit drinks and juices are full of sugar. Stop.

Diet sodas—they're also sweet, so get rid of them.

I know many of you'll hate me for this, but I'm not writing this book to lie to you.

David S. Ludwig, MD, PhD recently published an article in the Journal of the American Medical Association condemning artificial sweeteners. They interfere with your body's normal reaction to sugar, making your crave even more sweet foods. Another study found the more diet soda people drank, the more obese they were.

If you research aspartame online you'll find accusations that make the above paragraph look nice.

I don't pretend to know all the health risks of drinking either regular soda or diet soda.

I don't have to.

They help make or keep you fat and they're bad for your health.

That's enough to know. Don't drink them.

You know what to drink—plain water.

And what if you eat or drink something you know you "shouldn't?"

Take it easy, the world won't end, the sky won't fall and you won't even go to Purgatory, let alone Hell.

Chapter Five

Don't Deprive Yourself of Anything Except Guilt

I've never figured out why so many women want to equate food, sex and sin.

As in saying something such as, "This chocolate fudge sundae is so good it's positively sinful."

(I say women because I don't remember hearing any men say such things. Maybe it's because they have other sins on their minds. They certainly enjoy overeating also, but they seem to accept it as a natural part of life more than women do.)

Maybe it's just my warped view of religion. I wasn't brought up to think of things that made me feel good (such as—especially—sex) as sinful.

I've been sinful, but it was by hurting my friends and family.

So I don't think of overeating or eating high-sugar or high-carb foods (I also refuse to call such foods "bad") as sinful.

So, look, let's keep religion out of this. Believe what you want about God, the afterlife and what restrictions you should or needn't obey.

This book is about weight loss, not theology.

Eating foods that tend to make you overweight won't send you to Hell after you die—but they do tend to pack more fat into your fat cells.

That's isn't "bad" in a religious sense, but neither is it "good"—in any sense of the word.

I want you to forget about the religious words such as sin in relation to food because I also want you to forget another religious word in relation to food—guilt.

Save Your Guilt for Real Sins, Not for Food

Overeating or eating high-sugar or high-carb foods is not sinful, so there's no reason for you to feel guilty.

I'd say if eating a chocolate milkshake every night is the biggest "sin" you ever commit, you're a candidate for sainthood.

Face it—sometime in the future, you're going to eat something not on the approved list of foods on your eating plan. Or simply too much food.

Maybe tomorrow.

Maybe next week.

Maybe tonight.

It happens. Get over it.

Relax, take it easy, and forget about it.

Move on.

It's a mistake, not a sin.

It's a momentary, temporary movement away from your weight loss goal, and it's now in the past.

If you hear a little voice inside yourself berating yourself...

If you feel a sick, emotional hollowness in your stomach...

(If you ate so much the sick feeling in your stomach is physical, you'll just have to take some Alka-Seltzer, lie down and wait for it to go away.)

If you see a picture of yourself as a worthless person for eating something not on your weight loss program...

Relax.

If that's hard for you, don't worry. It's the subject of a later chapter.

Tomorrow is another day. As soon as possible, resume your weight loss program.

When I say "relax," I mean really relax, not the garbage ways people mistakenly call "relaxation."

Chapter Six

"Relax" Doesn't Mean You Can Do Whatever You Want and Still Lose Weight

Sometimes you just have to rely on common sense.

I knew when I came up with this book's title many people would—deliberately—misunderstand.

Many people will lump the word "relax" in their minds with such activities as—

Hanging out with friends and family

Drinking alcohol

Watching TV

Surfing the Web

Smoking marijuana

Sitting around

And—(drum roll please)...last but not least—

OVEREATING

By now, you should realize I'm not claiming the laws of biology have been repealed and you can stuff your face full of pizza, beer, chocolate cake, ice cream, candy bars and soda while sitting in front of the TV or computer until 2 AM at night and expect to lose weight.

I've nothing against hanging out with friends and family, surfing the Web or even watching TV.

But you've got to understand when I say "relax to lose weight," I mean—RELAX!

It means many things. You can do away with the stress caused by standard diet programs—

Counting the calories in the foods you eat

Adding up the calories you ate all day long

Adding up how many steps you took all day (some people actually do this) or how many calories you burned up through aerobic exercise

Keeping a food and diet journal or blog

Going to meetings

Tricking yourself by putting your dinner on a super small plate so the food looks bigger than it actually is. (My stomach was never fooled.)

You also get to do away with the stress caused by—

Carrying heavy grocery bags.

Buying expensive foods.

Sitting in fast food drive-through lanes

Walking into the gas station after you've already paid for your gas at the tank, because you need to spend extra money on soda and candy.

Thinking about how much money you throw away every week on empty calories and how much money you'd have if you simply put that into a savings account instead.

Watching grossly obese people shuffle up to a counter and realize you're buying even more snack food than they are. And of wondering how you look to thin people.

Not fitting into the largest size dress or slacks in the store.

Feeling your husband or lover turn over in bed every night, after just a goodnight peck.

Entering a bar or party, seeing men's heads turn toward you, give you a quick glance—and then turn their eyes away.

Fearing high blood pressure and diabetes, or the medicines you're already taking for those diseases.

Stuffing yourself until your stomach bulges so you can hardly move.

Instead of experiencing all that stress, I want you to just... plain...relax.

Is that too much to ask?

Instead of walking to the refrigerator for a beer or bowl of ice cream, relax and continue sitting on the coach.

Instead of fixing a big meal for yourself, relax and cook just enough.

Instead of staying up until one in the morning, relax and go to bed.

My hope for you is to eliminate all that stress from your life.

Relax—to lose weight.

You can start with your next breath.

Chapter Seven

Deep Breathing Starts You Burning Fat

We've established the connection between overweight and stress. Now we begin discovering a way to reduce stress so we lose that excess weight on our bodies.

It's a terrific break for your mind and body, and takes only about five minutes.

Not only that, it—

1. Gives you more energy.

2. Improves your digestion.

It helps you get more value from the nutrition in the food you do eat, so your body is less likely to feel undernourished, which pushes you to eat too much.

3. Makes your metabolism more efficient.

You'll burn more calories even while sitting at your computer or watching TV.

4. Improves your general health.

5. Burns calories even though you're barely moving.

6. Helps you relax and reduces your stress level.

7. Helps keep your spine limber.

8. Signals your pituitary gland to release endorphins into your nervous system.

Endorphins are the natural body chemicals that make you feel good when you eat chocolate and have sex. In fact, opiate drugs work by filling the endorphin receptors in your brain.

So this weight loss method actually gets you high—but is not addicting.

You can practice it anytime, anyplace. Including on the job in front of a computer screen or an angry customer or your boss.

Not only that, it's 100% free! No pills, no shakes, no monthly memberships, no equipment or uniform needed.

This wonderful health and weight loss technique is...

Slow, deep breathing.

Your brain, your heart, your lungs, your muscles and all the trillions of cells in your body will love you for it.

Few people breathe in a healthy manner. We tend to breathe too fast, too shallowly, too often and with our mouths open.

Since you're overweight, it's almost a certainty you fall into that category. It's even likely you breathe in ways even less healthy than most people, including while you sleep. (Most people with sleep apnea are overweight.)

The more you make a habit of slow, deep breathing, the healthier you are and the more weight you'll lose.

If Oxygen Were a New Drug, We'd Need a Prescription and It Would Cost a Fortune

The major fuel for our bodies is not food at all. It's not even water—it's oxygen.

Our cells convert oxygen into energy to use the food and water we consume. We need oxygen to think, to move, to digest food, to eliminate dead cells and to burn fat. 70% of our body's wastes such as dead cells and carbon dioxide are eliminated (or the body attempts to eliminate them) through our lungs, during exhalation.

Don't exhale fully, and you're aerobically and metabolically constipated. The toxins have to go somewhere, and so they do—into your fat cells.

And not getting enough oxygen signals your body to store fat instead of burning it for another reason. It takes oxygen to burn fat. If you're breathing shallowly, taking in barely enough oxygen to run your brain (which needs 20% of your total oxygen supply) and keep your other vital organs functioning, it figures it can't "afford" to spend oxygen to burn fat.

When you breathe deeply on a regular basis, your body comes to realize it now has enough oxygen to not only think and digest food, but to burn stored fat as well.

Plus, oxygen is the one thing we need our bodies can't store. We need a steady supply.

Yet so many people breath like it's not important. Stop taking oxygen for granted.

It's Your Oxygen—Suck It In

However, although as adults our lungs hold two gallons of air, most of us inhale only two or three pints. We settle for some air in our upper lungs instead of filling them completely, from the bottom.

If you bought a fountain soda like you breathe, you'd pay full price for a thirty-two ounce cup but fill only the bottom fourth with soda.

You'd never do that with a soda, so why do it with oxygen?

The way we can change our habitual, constant breathing practices is to sometimes be aware of them (we certainly can't all the time) and to make a habit of taking a few minutes daily to breathe deeply.

One problem is, for reasons I can't figure out even though I did the same thing as a child, most people think "deep breathing" means lifting our chests and sucking in air through our mouths.

This can help athletes rev themselves up before a competition, but it won't help calm you down or lose weight.

"Slow" deep breathing means, first of all, breathing slowwwwwwwly.

Not excruciatingly slow like a hibernating bear, but at a comfortable, deliberate pace.

Take three to five seconds to inhale.

Myself, I like to use four. If you're smaller or need to build up your lung capacity, use three. If you're in better shape than I— five.

Slow, "deep" breathing means, secondly, breathing deeply.

Hitching up your shoulders and chest is just the opposite.

The deep part of your lungs are at the bottom of your ribcage. You breathe deeply by expanding your stomach and diaphragm so air can start by filling up the bottom of your lungs. Then let your lungs ripple up, so the incoming air fills the middle of your lungs, then the top.

During our daily lives, most of us breath shallowly, using only the tops of our lungs. That's why we don't take in enough oxygen to stay thin, healthy and energetic.

Here's the Procedure:

It's easiest to sit comfortably (though you can stand too).

Keep your spine comfortably erect. If you tilt forward, you're squeezing your lungs, reducing their capacity.

Relax your belly muscles and diaphragm, letting them expand out.

(Yes, you read correctly—let your stomach swell. If you put your palm on your tummy you should feel it relax and move outward a little bit when you begin to inhale. Just as though there's a balloon just below your navel. If you can't you're not doing this correctly, and that may be one major reason you're carrying excess weight. Your body doesn't have enough oxygen to burn that fat.

So, just practice relaxing those muscles and letting them move out while you inhale. You can practice this by lying down flat on your back and putting a book on your stomach. Then practice raising the book when you begin to inhale. It can feel weird at first, but oddly relaxing.)

Inhale through your nose for three to four seconds, filling your lungs from bottom to top.

(Except during special breathing exercises as practiced by some disciplines such as yoga, or when you're breathing hard because you've just run two miles, you should breathe in and out through your nose, not your mouth.

(If evolution or God wanted us to breathe through our mouths, we wouldn't have noses.)

Hold for quadruple the time you spent inhaling. If you inhale for four seconds, hold for sixteen.

Exhale through your nose for double the inhalation time. If you inhale for four seconds and hold for sixteen, exhale for eight.

Repeat for a total of 10 times.

If you lose track (and it's amazing how quickly you feel so good and relaxed you can barely keep track of the number of repetitions), don't sweat it. One more or less will not break you.

Do a set of ten in the morning, the middle of the day and at night.

Many people have lost weight doing nothing but that.

Breathe Deeply Whenever You're Tempted to Feel Bored

Pay attention to your breathing during the rest of your life.

When you need to be at a mental peak—say you're drafting an important report at work—start out by taking 10 slow deep breaths. Your brain will appreciate the extra oxygen and reward you with additional insights and ideas.

During and after a long spell of work, take a few deep breaths. If you can't work in all ten, that's OK. One is enough to 95% relax you and give you the energy to go on.

Whenever you feel stressed out by a customer, a client, a co-worker, your boss, traffic, your husband, or your kids...notice you're probably holding your breath.

Relax and let it out. Take a slow, deep breath. That won't make the problem go away, but it will give you the chance to think of a more helpful response than either crying or screaming.

One warning. If you take a slow deep breath at a long red light or while stuck in a long line of traffic, the light will turn green or the car in front of you will move forward, interrupting your relaxing breath.

Which will irritate you.

But hey, at least you're moving again!

Deep breathing is also a good way to spend your time while you're waiting in line at the bank or supermarket, during a boring meeting or presentation on the job, or while you wait for your computer to finish some automatic systems thing it does when you need to check your email.

It's also great while you're watching TV.

At such times you don't have to hold your breath, just inhale deeply and exhale, practicing filling your lungs with good old-fashioned—even free!—oxygen.

Many indoor environments with air conditioning don't have as much oxygen as the outside air. All the more reason to fill your lungs so you can inhale as much oxygen as possible.

Breathe Deeply Instead of Eating Unhealthy Food

Add eating unhealthy food to that list of stressors.

See a billboard for McDonald's that makes you salivate like Pavlov's dog? Take a slow deep breath.

Pay for your gas and suddenly feel thirsty because you see somebody carrying two extra-large glasses of soda? Take a slow deep breath.

Go into your office break room and find a large cake for somebody's birthday? Take a slow deep breath.

Watch a movie late at night and suddenly crave a bowl of chocolate fudge ice cream? Take a slow deep breath. Heck, take two. Take three.

This book is about relaxing to lose weight. So, relax already.

In case you've forgotten (and chances are good that you have), that's what the next chapter is about.

Chapter Eight

The Easy Way to Take It Easy

Many years ago I was friends with a girl studying to become a physical therapist. I'd been practicing yoga since I was twelve, including the resting asana fondly called the "corpse," but she taught me something I'd never known.

The deepest, best relaxation comes after intense strain.

This seems incredible, but she held my leg while I tried to lift it as hard as I could, and then I stopped.

It felt terrific.

My leg muscles melted into the floor.

Years later, I read advice to combine this with the yoga asana by systematically tensing, then relaxing, all muscles in the body from toes to top of head. That greatly helped me benefit from that motionless yoga posture.

There are a thousand variations of this. Some start with physical relaxation as I just did. Many others start with the mind, calling it meditation.

Herbert Benson made this popular in 1975 with his book THE RELAXATION RESPONSE. He advises simply sitting comfortably, relaxing, then focusing your mind on a meaningless sound or image. Nothing mystic or exciting—just something neutral or peaceful to keep remembering when your mind drifts off into other thoughts, as it will.

Meditation is Total Relaxation, Total Relaxation is Meditation

Hindus use the sound of "om" or other mantras. Some disciplines advocates picturing a lotus blossom, rose or candle flame.

Jose Silva connected this to new research on brain waves. He found people could quickly learn to train their brains to emit mostly alpha waves, as we do when on the verge of sleeping. Other people use self-hypnosis.

After relaxing your muscles through systematically tensing them, take ten or so slow, deep breaths. This will also help you to relax physically and mentally.

Some people sit on the floor with crossed legs, others in a comfortable chair.

I learned from yoga to lie flat on the floor. Some say it's too easy in this position to fall asleep. I say—so what? If I fall asleep it must be because I needed the rest.

Many techniques suggest imagining yourself in a special place in your mind. Some people like to feel themselves at a tropical beach. Others go to a beautiful pasture. Others feel sheltered in a deep underground cave or in space ship.

Whatever works for you, works. There're no rules, only suggestions to play with.

Do what feels good. Relaxation is its own reward.

If you want some help or guidance, there're a thousand CDs for sale online that will induce a state of relaxation. Search for Silva method, self-hypnosis, alpha waves, guided imagery, and meditation.

You can spend a small fortune on them if you wish, but you really only need one good one. Play it while wearing a set of quality headphones.

And you actually don't need any CDs. Holy men and women—and many not so holy—meditated for tens of thousands of years before the invention of recorded sound.

Practice this meditation or relaxation for ten to fifteen minutes a day, at least once or twice a day. Two times is even better, and three times is most excellent.

Now Try a Technique I'm Stealing From the Silva Method

Once you've entered a state of deep physical, mental and emotional relaxation, put the tips of your thumbs and forefingers together.

After you've done that a few times, you've trained yourself to associate the act of touching your thumb tips to your forefinger tips with that state of deeply profound relaxation.

This is called a trigger or anchor—and it has many uses.

Reinforce this trigger every time you meditate.

Meditating this way will naturally reduce your cortisol and help you lose weight and just plain feel better.

However, once we feel comfortable in that state, we can use its power to change our lives, including losing weight permanently.

Because thin people are thin, and in this state we can transform ourselves into thin people.

Chapter Nine

The Thin You Starts in Your Mind

This is the most important chapter of this book. If you read and practice what's in this chapter, you'll lose weight and keep it off even if you don't read the rest of the book.

This is the heart of permanent weight-loss. The information in the other chapters will make it easier, and your particular eating plan can affect it, but in the end your results depend on how you see yourself.

Now you've learned the importance of controlling stress, the importance of breathing deeply and how to relax and meditate, now you can use that state of relaxation and meditation to change your self-image.

Your Self-Image is More Powerful Than Surgery and Mirrors

Self-image psychology was popularized back in 1960 with publication of the book PSYCHO-CYBERNETICs by Dr. Maxwell Maltz. Maltz was a plastic surgeon who noticed something in his practice that puzzled him.

Sometimes after he repaired or improved someone's face, they insisted he'd done nothing. Their nose was still too big. That big scar still marred their cheek.

That led him to wonder why those patients didn't or couldn't accept what everybody else could see and what every mirror reflected back to them—their faces did look different.

Many of these patients admitted the mirror showed their nose was now smaller, then insisted the mirror was wrong!

He eventually discovered although he could repair physical faces, some patients didn't change their inner self-images to match their new features.

Further research led Dr. Maltz to realize we all have self-images that control not only whether we believe we're beautiful or ugly, but whether we believe we're smart or stupid, fat or thin, good or bad mothers, good or bad at our jobs, and so on.

It's difficult for us to do anything that goes against our self-image.

You Can Do Everything You Decide To See Yourself Doing

For example, what is the difference between me and a mountain climber?

It's not physical conditioning. I'm not as strong as they are, but if I saw myself as a mountain climber I'd begin working out a lot more.

It's not knowledge. If I saw myself as a mountain climber, I'd begin learning about ropes and pylons.

It's not experience. Every mountain climber had to climb their first mountain.

It's just I don't see myself as a mountain climber. I don't want to be a mountain climber. But you know what? If I wanted to climb mountains, I'd begin preparing for that and eventually I'd climb a mountain or ten.

If you want to be thin— and especially if you want to remain thin—you must think of yourself as thin person. You must see yourself inside your mind as a thin person.

Sure, maybe you're fifty or a hundred pounds heavier than your ideal thin weight—right now.

But "right now" will be in the past by the time you finish reading this chapter.

Here's Something to Think About

Think about your best friend or family member who's so thin you're jealous of her.

Now, just imagine this—what would happen if tonight a magic genie transferred all your excess fat from your body to hers?

If you continue to think of yourself as "fat," (even though that's no longer objectively true), you'll continue to eat too much and too many sugar-rich and carb-rich foods and not exercise enough.

It'll take time, but eventually, if you refuse to change your self-image, you'll regain the weight.

And your thin friend? She has a "thin" self-image, so she'll continue to eat just enough healthy food and to remain active.

It'll take time, but she'll lose that weight.

(By the way, do you think she'd start going to weekly meetings, counting calories, keeping a food journal or blog or buy smaller plates? No, she'd just continue to eat and act like a thin person.

(That's another reason I don't like all that claptrap—they're things only "fat" people do. You'll lose more weight by acting like a thin person and doing the things thin people do.)

In a few years, if neither one of you change your self-images, you'll be overweight again and she'll be thin again.

Make the Thin You More Powerful and Compelling Every Time You Breathe Deeply and Relax

Fortunately, you can change your self-image.

When you spend ten or twenty minutes relaxing or meditating, once or thrice a day, now you have a purpose.

Instead of concentrating on some sound or image, you think about yourself—as a thin person.

See yourself as thin. How do you look at your ideal weight? See yourself there.

See yourself in summer clothes, a bikini, in underwear, in your job's uniform or business clothes, in a sexy party dress, and naked.

See yourself at all your usual activities, and doing things you'd like to do but now avoid because of your weight. Gardening, dancing, walking through the park—see yourself thin and gorgeous.

See yourself as sexually attractive. See them lusting after you ("them" can be your husband/boyfriend, many men or many women—it's up to you).

And your clothes? Nothing you wear now. You're either in one of those outfits you used to wear but which are now hanging in the back of your closet, or something brand new in your new, thin size.

Feel the energy, the tingling feeling of a healthy slim body in super health. Just imagine how great it feels to be thin and healthy.

Just Keep on Seeing Yourself Easily Eating Only Healthy Foods

And hear yourself saying things such as "It's so great to feel thin. I don't need a soda, just a bottle of water please. No dessert for me. I have enough energy to climb a mountain. It was so easy. I just realized I didn't want to eat fattening foods anymore. Chocolate pie is not sinful—it's just extra calories I don't need or want."

Hear the people around you saying things such as, "You look terrific. Congratulations. It's like you're a new person now."

Make the pictures big, bright and moving like an ultra-large 3-D movie. The sounds are crisp, loud and pleasant. The feeling is intense ecstasy.

Magnify all these experiences. Make them bigger, stronger, brighter—a million times more powerful until you're overwhelmed by the wonderful intensity of how great it is to be the thin you.

Hug all that to yourself, folding it to your chest so you feel it all inside you.

Because, after all, it IS you. You're that thin woman.

Yes, your body still has to lose a few pounds. But inside—where it counts the most—you ARE that thin woman.

And remember to touch your thumb to your forefinger to anchor those terrific sensations.

That way, you can relive that wonderful state of thinness even when faced with the real world.

Chapter Ten

Blowing Out Your Fat Anchors

When you take slow deep breaths, relax physically and live through your thin self-image mind-movies with the tip of your index finger against the tip of your thumb, you've establishing that gesture as what's called an anchor or trigger.

Touch your fore finger to your thumb and you breathe deeply, relax and remind yourself that you're a thin person—re-experiencing the pleasure and energy of the thin you.

You can regain this state even during your daily life.

Whenever you're stressed out.

Especially whenever you start to feel a craving to eat a food not on your eating program or simply too much food.

Establish the habit of doing this throughout your day (and night) as stressful and potential overweight situations come up.

Establish the habit of doing this in the aftermath of stressful situations (for example, a difficult meeting with your boss), when you feel like "rewarding" yourself with a candy bar or something similar.

Instead, reward yourself with increased oxygen, luxurious

relaxation and a reminder of how wonderful it feels to be thin.

Practice in private, in one of your daily sessions.

Keep Living Through Mental Movies of the Thin You Now Indifferent to Unhealthy Food

After you breathe deeply 10 times and physically relax, think of all the situations where you commonly eat like a "fat" person—and then in your mind see your inner thin self react like a thin person.

You're pushing your shopping cart through the supermarket past the baked goods display. Is that a signal to you to buy some doughnuts and sweet rolls?

Watch your thin self push the cart right past that section. Feel her indifference. Hear her say to herself, "The canned tomatoes are on sale."

Your kids demand a visit to the Golden Arches. For their sake, you give in. For yourself, you order only a salad and glass of water.

It's four o'clock. You're finally getting your afternoon break. The customers are driving you crazy. So are your co-workers. You're tired. Your nerves are frazzled. Your blood sugar has evaporated. If you don't eat something soon, you're sure to drop dead before you can drive home. The chips and snack cakes in the vending machines are singing out your name.

You see yourself ignore the machines and pull out a cup of vanilla yogurt.

You're at a party. It's late Saturday night. The pizza slices sit right next to the big bowl of M&Ms which sit right next to the burritos which sit right next to the huge sub sandwich which sits right next to the cans of beer and soda.

You watch yourself take a slice of sandwich, eat only the lettuce, cheese and meat in the middle, wash it down with bottled water and throw the bread slices away.

You're watching TV late at night. The movie is still an hour from its suspenseful conclusion. A fast food commercial airs. All of a sudden you want to call and order a pepperoni pizza.

You watch yourself get off the couch, walk to the refrigerator and pull out a few pieces of string cheese and an apple.

You get the idea.

Systematically Live Through Every Possible Real Life Scenario, Changing It to the Thin You

Make a list of the times and places where you habitually overeat. Whether it's visiting Aunt Nelly or waiting for an airplane or just going to Burger King because you've been eating dinner there every Wednesday for twenty years.

Then, in your mind, live through those situations, and meet them as the thin you.

Maybe you take have to take a few nibbles to be polite. OK, it happens. Don't sweat it.

Many situations can be avoided just by keeping your mind on other things. Don't notice the billboards. Don't pay attention to the print ads and commercials. Don't listen to the radio blurbs. Drive right by the fast food joints. Confine your grocery shopping to the healthy sections of the supermarket.

Watching TV or chatting online? Focus on the movie or the website—forget about food.

The Next Step: Meet Those Situations For Real and GET IN THEIR FACE!

First of all, practice the above for at least a month. Move on to this step only after you feel 100% sure the real, new thin you is indifferent to these signals.

Now, you did all of the above in your imagination, in the inner theater of your mind.

But real life is real, isn't it?

So, for at least the next three days—longer if you feel the need—deliberately meet as many of these situations as you can.

Step one—allow yourself to feel that desire, that absolute craving, as deeply as you can. Absorb it, live it, drown in the desire for sugar, for fat, for cakes and pies and beer and pizza and Cokes and Mountain Dews and Krispy Kreme doughnuts.

Step Two. At the peak of your lust for sugar or Fritos—just before you give in to your desires—put your finger and thumb together.

Step Three. The desire for unhealthy food vanishes. Breathe slowly and deeply, relaxed, and experience your thin self.

It's as Easy as One-Two-Three to Change How You React to Food and Food Marketing

That billboard making you daydream about burrito supremes?

Let it!

Mmm, ground beef, tomatoes and sour cream with taco sauce. Yum yum!

Forefinger and thumb together. The thin you is indifferent. She just keeps on planning a game to play with her kids after dinner.

Go up to the vending machines in your workplace break room. Look at all those bags of potato chips, snack cakes and candy bars.

Go, look them right in the eye! You can taste them right now. Crispy, luscious, delicious.

Then put your thumb and forefinger together and feel your thin self's thoughts. She just reminds herself of the importance of taking healthy snacks to work every morning.

Need to fill your gas tank? Go into the station and look a long look around at the rows of candy bars, cakes, doughnuts, sandwiches, and other snacks.

Wouldn't they all taste great? Go on, salivate all you want.

Then put your thumb and forefinger together. Let your thin self remember she's in there only to pay for her gasoline. She gives the attendant the money and walks out.

And don't forget to practice this during the really hard situations.

The times you eat restricted foods because you're lonely.

Or depressed.

Or frustrated.

Or angry at the world and yourself.

These are the most difficult because it seems as though obesity is not your main problem. Your personal problem, whatever it is, is your real problem.

And that's undoubtedly true.

If You Need Professional Help for Other Issues, Get It

I can't make your personal problems disappear, much as I'd like to. We all go through bad times and get the blues.

If yours are serious, get professional help. Or at least talk things out with your friends and family.

But as your Relax to Lose Weight Program coach, I'm here to tell you two things.

1. Whatever else is wrong in your life, becoming or remaining overweight will NOT help you.

Most likely, you'll use your weight as one more reason to feel bad about yourself. That's the last thing you need, for your physical and emotional health.

2. You can break the habitual link you've probably formed

between feeling emotionally bad and overeating in an unhealthy attempt to feel better.

So do the above practice with your emotional states. However, use common sense. If you have a problem with depression, do NOT go all the way into feeling bad. Simply remember what it feels like, then touch your finger and thumb together, take slow and deep breaths, relax and call your thin self-image to mind.

See yourself dealing with your other problems in a constructive way (including getting professional help if you need). This does NOT include scarfing down an entire chocolate cake!

I recommend going through this procedure for every "fat" time in your daily life. You know when they are. I've given typical scenarios as examples. You know which ones apply to you.

Go through them all—day after day...

Until it becomes a habit to act like your inner, thin self-image.

Pretty soon you won't think about it all. It'll be automatic.

As soon as you glimpse a billboard for your favorite fast food restaurant, you'll automatically take a deep breath, relax and picture yourself as thin.

After a little time and practice, this will happen so fast you won't even notice, you'll just keep on driving and listening to the radio.

You'll be acting thin and you won't even miss a beat.

Good job!

But what about the days you're "allowed" to "cheat" on your

diet?

Or the plateaus when the weight stops coming off no matter what you do?

Chapter Eleven

Plateaus and Cheat Days

Remember our bodies evolved under much different conditions that exist in the developed world today.

Until just recently, food was scarce for almost everybody alive most of the time.

Men had to go out hunting, risking their lives to track and run down game. Or they waded into rivers with spears to catch fish.

Women spent a lot of time walking around, foraging leaves and roots. In season they gathered fruits and berries.

Sometimes game was scarce. During winter—and the Ice Ages were mainly winter—there was hardly any plants or animals around to eat.

When they came across a tree of ripe fruit, they stuffed themselves.

When they killed a mastodon, they stuffed themselves.

When they found a beach full of crabs, they stuffed themselves.

And the people who could store that food in their bodies the longest were most likely to survive the long cruel winters.

Our bodies evolved complex ways to prevent weight loss, for fear of starvation.

The 10% Then Plateau Rule

We can lose the first 10% pretty easily. So if you now weigh 200 pounds, a good diet and exercise program will get you down to 180 in a few months.

However, after that your body's defense mechanisms kick in.

Oh oh, your body thinks. The food supply is low. I need to kick in some conservation methods or we'll die of starvation.

We don't even know everything the body does, but for weeks or months, no matter how little you eat or how much you exercise, you'll lose little or no weight.

You just have to accept progress will not be linear. You'll have ups and downs.

Eventually, however, if you keep on your new program, your body will get the message.

Hey, 180 pounds is OK, it eventually decides. I've been that weight for the past two months and haven't died of starvation. It's the new normal, so I can go back to normal functioning.

Then you start losing weight again. Once you've lost another 18 pounds or so (10% of your new-normal weight), you'll hit a plateau again.

Just get used to the idea.

Cheat Days—Meals are Better—Can Raise Your Levels of Leptin

I used to believe cheat days were just somebody's goofy idea to justify eating what they knew they shouldn't. Then I read about the hormone leptin, which controls how fat you feel.

Not only that, leptin can help you get through those plateaus, because it's one of the feedback mechanisms your body has in place to prevent starvation.

Leptin controls how much fat you burn.

When your body has high levels of leptin, you burn more fat.

Low levels of leptin? You don't burn fat.

And what lowers your levels of leptin?

For one thing, eating a low number of calories.

So when you reduce the amount of food you eat over time, even though you're eating more sensibly, your body responds by lowering leptin.

Which lowers your ability to burn fat.

So how can you keep leptin levels high?

That's where "cheat days" come in. One day a week, or one meal of one day a week, you eat a meal high in calories.

Hey, I'm not starving after all! your body thinks. So it's safe to go back to higher levels of leptin and burning fat.

This doesn't mean go crazy by eating a large pepperoni pizza, washing it down with beer and having a cake for dessert.

It does mean eating larger portions of good food so you take in plenty of calories so your body understands you're not about to starve to death during an Ice Age winter stuck in a cave.

Also—and nobody likes to talk about this—once you do reach your ideal weight, there's no more need for cheat days. You eat just enough to maintain good health at your ideal weight.

Don't forget to drink a glass of water too.

Chapter Twelve

Water - Drink Your Fill

What's the easiest thing to drink when you're thirsty?

I'll give you a hint. You don't have to open a can. It may come in a bottle, but is just as far away as a drinking fountain or a faucet.

Yes, of course it's water. And most people don't drink enough. And it does affect your ability to lose weight—for many reasons.

1. One thing that can keep you feeling hungry is undernourishment of your body. Your cells crave the vitamins and minerals they need to function in a healthy manner. When they feel deprived, YOU feel deprived, so you grab something to eat to fill the vacuum.

If you grab a candy bar, you're obviously not giving your cells the nourishment they need and want.

It's less obvious, but if you don't drink enough water, you can eat a plate of a superfood such as green algae and yet your cells won't benefit much because your blood can't squeeze through your capillaries to deliver the supernutrition you just ate.

You want your blood to flow freely to perform its many important functions, including bringing nutrition to your cells. When you're dehydrated your blood is thick and sluggish.

2. Blood also delivers oxygen to your cells. Your cells can't operate well without enough oxygen. They feel tired and run down. They don't operate at full strength. This means they're not burning the calories they should be burning, and you don't feel healthy.

You're not as healthy, because your cells perform important functions. When they're operating at a subpar level, so do you.

Plus, that fatigue either keeps you from healthy exercise and/or makes you feel like eating something you know you shouldn't, just because you know sugar and/or caffeine will give you a jolt of energy.

3. Have you ever gotten angry with a co-worker because you had to back them up so much you couldn't perform your own job functions?

It's a common complaint in many workplace break rooms around the world.

When you don't drink enough water, you're placing the same burden on your poor liver, and it's weight loss that pays the price.

See, it's your kidneys' job to filter waste products from your blood. They need a lot of water to do that. When you're dehydrated, they can't function optimally.

But your body MUST get rid of those waste products, or you begin dying. So when your kidneys are low on water, your liver has to back them up.

So what?

It's your liver's job to convert stored fat into energy. When it's busy covering for your kidneys because they don't have enough water to do their job, your liver doesn't have time or energy to convert stores of fat into energy.

Your liver would probably gripe about your kidneys if it could but, let's face it, if you're not drinking enough water it's your fault you're not losing weight.

4. When you do burn those calories, the oxidation process creates more waste products. You need to flush them out of your body for simple good health.

When you feel an urge to eat or drink something, just because you feel like eating or drinking something but you're not really hungry, satisfy yourself with water.

After Breathing Deeply, Drinking Lot of Water is the Healthiest Thing You Can do

Drink a glass of water before a meal and you'll eat less.

Drinking water could also help other health problems.

For instance, making your blood flow better helps prevent and relieve headaches.

Drinking lots of water reduces your risk of kidney stones.

Drinking lots of water also helps prevent high blood pressure.

That may sound odd, but it really makes sense. When you don't drink enough water, your body wants to hang on to what it has.

This is similar to what happens when you go on a starvation

diet. You lose weight at first, but then your body starts doing everything it can to hang on to your fat, so you don't starve to death.

When you don't drink enough water, your body doesn't want to let go of water, so it retains it in your flesh. That's why so many overweight people have such flabby lower arms, swollen legs and puffy ankles.

However, once you start drink ample water, your body starts getting rid of the excess water in your tissues, so you establish a healthy balance of water going in and out.

I've seen weight loss experts advise drinking ice cold water so your body will burn calories to warm it up.

That sounds to me like just another ridiculous gimmick. I say, drink it cold, cool or hot—whatever you like. But drink lots more of if than you already are.

Drink it one glass at a time, through your day. You can't absorb more than eight to ten ounces at one time.

Stop drinking three to four hours before you go to bed unless you enjoy getting up in the middle of the night to stumble to the bath room.

Don't go to any trouble to pop open a car of soda or beer, or coffee or tea or juice or lemonade or an energy drink or a fruit drink.

Take the easy way—drink water.

Speaking of bedtime...

Chapter Thirteen

Sleep More, Weigh Less

The most extreme form of relaxation is sleep.

Therefore, getting plenty of sleep every night is an important part of the "Relax to Lose Weight" Program.

From 1986 to 1994 researchers followed over 68,000 women. It's a famous project called The Nurses Health Study. Over those sixteen years, many of the women gained weight (no surprise there!), but women who reported getting less than five hours sleep gained more weight than those who got at least seven hours a night. This was true despite physical activity and diet.

There was a clear connection: the less a woman slept, the more weight she gained.

Other studies have established the connection in both children and adults. People who sleep less than seven hours a night are more likely to be obese.

Scientists don't agree on exactly why this is true.

Common sense tells us people who go to bed earlier don't eat as much late at night. It's also possible women who haven't slept enough are too tired to be physically active during the day.

And most of us understand there's a connection between daytime fatigue and overeating. I can't count how many candy bars I've bought from the vending machine at work because I felt so tired (but of course couldn't take a nap because I was on the job.).

Let the Thin You Dream Sweet Dreams

It could also be women staying up late at night are also taking in other substances that affect their sleep: alcohol, tobacco, and marijuana. Many people with these habits tend to snack a lot. And of course, alcohol is its own source of excess calories.

Sleep deprivation also affects important hormones, such as ghrelin and leptin. These two hormones act together. Leptin makes you feel full. Ghrelin makes you feel hungry.

Because not getting enough sleep reduces levels of leptin and increases levels of ghrelin, it's hardly surprising sleep-deprived people eat more.

And in studies done by the University of Illinois in Chicago and at Stanford University in California, sleep-deprived, low-leptin high-ghrelin volunteers also craved mostly high carbohydrate, calorie-dense food.

There's also reason to believe not getting enough sleep lowers basal metabolic rate.

That is how your body runs normally from moment to moment— heart beat, breathing, blood flowing and so on.

The higher your metabolic rate, the more calories you burn— even while you're sleeping or while you're sitting in front of your computer hardly moving.

Some researchers—and all of us in our daily lives—have noticed a connection between stress and sleep loss.

When we're depressed or upset, we can't sleep well if we do go to bed, so we stay up watching TV or surfing the Net—and wind up eating something we wouldn't have if we'd gone to bed.

Increasing HGH Keeps Us Younger and Thinner

Another important hormone affects our weight—human growth hormone (HGH).

Human growth hormone is the closest thing we've found to the fountain of youth. The levels of HGH in our bodies control how old we are biologically, including our Body Mass Index (BMI)—a medical way of saying how fat we are.

The higher our HGH levels, the more lean body mass we have and the less fat we carry.

The higher our HGH levels, the more closer we are to being the slim trim sixteen years old we used to be.

HGH is manufactured in and secreted from our pituitary gland. Our pituitaries manufacture the same amount our entire lives, but for some reason release less as we grow older.

If you're over sixty years of age, your doctor is cooperative, you don't mind injecting yourself with a needle every day and you have about $2,000 per month of extra income, you can take the actual hormone.

For the rest of us, the usual ways of increasing HGH are:

1. Fasting (Some people do this and obviously it will help you lose weight, but it's too stressful for me.)

2. Intense exercise (I discuss this in a later chapter.)

3. Get more deep sleep

That's because 75% of our natural HGH is released during deep sleep. If you don't sleep at least seven hours per night, you're not getting enough deep sleep to keep your HGH levels at an optimum level.

The less HGH you have, the biologically older you are—and increased weight is one of the official signs of aging.

As a former pizza delivery driver, I know many people stay up late at night watching movies and sports—and eating pizza (and often drinking beer).

I hate to deprive your local delivery driver of your tips, but I strongly suggest you go to bed earlier—even on Saturday night.

Do get plenty of rest, because in the next chapter we start (easy) exercising.

Chapter Fourteen

The Final Key to Healthy Weight Loss—Exercise

Arggh!! I can hear some of you screaming.

I thought she said this was a "relax" to lose weight program? How can I relax while I'm jogging my brains out? I don't want to exercise.

Hey—relax.

Just as I'm not responsible for you confusing the word "relaxing" with "partying and eating too much," I'm not responsible for you thinking "relaxing" means ONLY sitting or lying motionless.

It can mean that, and that's great, and I've covered the motionless meditation thing.

But you can't sit or lie motionless all day long.

If you're following the program so far, you're creating a self-image of yourself as thin, healthy and energetic. You're eating moderate amounts of healthy foods. You're sleeping at least seven hours every night. You're taking 10 slow, deep breaths followed by deep relaxation one to three times a day. You're drinking lots of water.

You're dealing better with stressful situations in your life.

You're meeting daily weight loss challenges just as a thin person would—with courtesy and indifference.

Now you're happier, healthier, thinner—and have more energy than you know what to do with.

Hey, it's not relaxing to coop your body up when it's so stoked with passion and the joy of living.

However, running for miles is NOT what I'm asking you to do.

I also don't want you to lift weights, buy expensive exercise equipment or join a gymnasium.

I believe in relaxing exercise.

Let's start with the easiest kind—walking.

Chapter Fifteen

Walk and Lose Weight

You've probably heard about the many health benefits of walking. You've seen people walking around malls. You've seen them in their neighborhoods and in parks.

You may not have heard walking is the most common exercise of people registered with the National Weight Control Registry which follows people who have lost at least 30 pounds and kept it off for at least one year.

The Diabetes Prevention Program found walking at least 150 minutes a week plus reducing body fat by 5% reduced the risk of diabetes by 58%.

Research even connects walking with reduced risk of breast and colon cancer. Women who walked from 1.25 hours to 2.5 hours per week had 18% less breast cancer. Other studies have connected walking with less risk of colon cancer.

And when I write walking, I mean simple walking. Wear a comfortable pair of shoes, comfortable clothes for the weather and go.

Don't Complicate the Simplest Exercise of All

I don't advocate wearing extra weights, listening to the radio or a CD or walking at high speed as though you can't wait to finish. I don't take a pedometer to count my steps. I don't use a gadget to monitor my heart beat.

If you enjoy walking with a buddy, that's great. Just don't get so attached to their company you don't walk when they're not available. Don't use them as an excuse not to walk.

Take your kids. Take your dog. Make it fun, and something you do on a regular basis.

Me, I love to just walk at a medium speed. I enjoy the plants and flowers, if any. I say hello to other people, though I don't stop to chat. I'm usually in a small park close to my home. I enjoy the sound of the ducks in the pond and the children playing.

Sometimes I think about my personal problems and what I need to do about them.

Sometimes I think about writing projects, and often get a lot of good ideas.

Sometimes I think about enjoyable people and events in my past. Sometimes I plan for the future. Sometimes I just enjoy remembering good movies. When I'm reading a good novel, I sometimes write scenes in my head the author skipped over.

By the time I return home, I feel physically, emotionally and mentally refreshed and rejuvenated. I have the ideas and energy to sit in front of my computer and write for hours.

Walking Fine-Tunes Your Body's Metabolism

One hour a day is my goal. Sometimes weather and circumstances keep me inside.

However, I advise you to also aim to walk an hour a day, at least five days a week. Every day is even better.

You'll burn a few calories while you walk, but what's more important is you'll be making your metabolism more efficient and healthier. That means you'll burn even more calories just living than if you hadn't taken that walk.

You'll burn more calories in the twenty-three hours between your walks than you will in the hour when you're actually walking.

The weight loss magic of exercise is not "burning" calories during the activity, it's in how much it improved your health and your metabolism during the rest of your day and night.

No huffing and puffing necessary.

It also does wonders for your mood. That's not just me talking, either. Research has found people who walk for thirty minutes, three to five times a week, have less depression. If you feel the need to eat to relax, take a walk instead.

It helps you keep thinking—researchers have discovered women who walk at least one and a half hours a week have better cognitive function (thinking) and less decline with age than women who walked less than forty minutes per week.

However, although it's the simplest and most accessible "Relax to Lose Weight Program" exercise, walking is not the only one.

Sometimes you need to move other parts of your bodies, in other directions, not to mention incorporating breathing, massaging your inner organs and increasing your supply of life energy.

Take a cue from ancient Hindus and Chinese, and Joseph Pilates.

Chapter Sixteen

Yoga, Qigong and Pilates

Walking is terrific basic exercise. If you can, however, I suggest you also spend time practicing a greater variety of physical movements.

I say "movements" rather than "exercise" because although these are systems called "exercise," they are NOT calisthenics or body weight exercises designed to build your muscles. They're not strenuous or exhausting. They have nothing to do with a lot of sweaty pushups.

They are gentle, slow and relaxing—just right for those who want to lose weight without a lot of exertion and strain.

They're best for shaping and balancing your body, improving posture, strengthening your inner organs, and re-energizing.

I can't say I practice them regularly or that I'm an expert, but I enjoy yoga, qigong and Pilates.

All three are fascinating, and a world unto themselves, though with a lot of crossover (Pilates incorporates some yoga. Yoga and qigong share some background, perhaps because their practice was spread back and forth between ancient India and China by traders or wandering monks.)

And all three have inspired many books by people who are experts.

This chapter can only be an introduction. I encourage you to read more books and invest in DVDs.

Pick the One That's Best for You

You don't have to try to do all three. That'd be too much. All three are excellent for overall health. I don't think anybody can claim one is "better" than the other.

Therefore, go with the one that seems best for you, or at least more convenient. Find out if anybody is giving classes in your town. I believe it'll be easier to find qualified yoga or Pilates instructors than qigong unless you're in a big city or close to a large Chinese neighborhood.

However, although it's recommended, at least at first, it's not necessary to go to classes—unless you have a physical condition requiring oversight by a teacher.

I read my first book on yoga when I was only twelve years old. I couldn't have gone to classes even if there'd been any (and in those days there probably wasn't). It didn't occur to me to care. I had a thick rug on my bedroom floor and enough open space to practice the asanas, and that's all I needed.

That's all you need too. Some open space, a little time and privacy. Some people buy yoga or Pilates mats. A thick carpet or rug works too. You need just enough to cushion your spine from a hard floor. A gymnastic or wrestling mat is perfect but not required.

I suggest keeping your area quiet and peaceful, or playing only relaxing, pleasant nonobstrusive music.

Hatha Yoga

Technically, there're many kinds of yoga. The goal of all of them is to reach a peak of religious experience and enlightenment. What we call just yoga is Hatha yoga and is considered the least important.

The goal of Hatha yoga is to improve a disciple's health so they can handle meditating for hours at a time without physical pain distracting them.

The first book I read was YOGA AND HEALTH by Selvarajan Yesudian and Elisabeth Haich. It was old even when I first read it, but sometimes it's still available on Amazon, where many agree it's still the best book on yoga.

Selvarajan was a sickly boy growing up even though his father was a Western-style doctor. When he was fifteen he started going to a yoga instructor and within several years was strong and healthy.

Yoga consists of three parts: physical postures (asanas), breathing exercises (pranayama) and total relaxation, which you've already learned.

The postures are not designed to increase your strength as calisthenics do, although some of them do take strength. They stretch and balance you. And yes, some of them twist you up in strange ways. That puts beneficial pressure on your inner organs, keeping them functioning well. It's like giving your liver a massage. And some of the most beneficial ones turn you upside down, improving blood flow to your brain.

As taught in this book, the postures are performed slowly and deliberately. Half the benefit lies in trying them, in making the effort to stretch and improve.

You should already be taking ten deep breaths three times a day. Pranayama will take you beyond that.

Part of the underlying theory is there's an elemental life force called "prana" in Sanskrit. The postures and breathing are to increase and balance our supplies of prana.

Qigong

Thousands of years ago when Indian monks were developing the Hatha yoga system, their counterparts in China were also coming up with movements and breathing for greater health.

You've probably seen pictures of large groups of Chinese people practicing qigong or t'ai chi in parks early in the morning.

Technically, they're doing t'ai chi, a form of martial arts, but the line between it and qigong is not clear.

Qigong consists of slow movements which somehow improve your strength, health, balance and coordination. And there are ways to breathe as you move—as well as sit and breathe and meditate.

The basic goal is to build up your supplies of the elemental life force called "qi" in Chinese. The movements and breathing increase and balance our supplies of qi.

Sound familiar? Yes, although there are philosophical and religious differences in how Indians explain yoga and how Chinese explain qigong, at their core they're similar.

For our superficial purposes, the main difference—in my opinion—is qigong is a lot more focused on movement. Yoga is more focused on getting your body into a position which you hold for a while. And while getting there smoothly is important, it's not the movement itself which is the point.

Pilates

Joseph Pilates was born in Germany in 1883. Even though his father was a gymnast and his mother a naturopath, he was sickly child suffering from asthma, rickets and rheumatic fever.

He started studying ways to train his body, including body building, gymnastics and yoga. By the age of fourteen he was posing for anatomy charts.

As a young man he worked as a gymnast, boxer, diver, circus performer and self-defense trainer, eventually moving from Germany to England.

This turned out to be a terrific career move. In 1914, because of World War I, the government of England interned him on the Isle of Man along with other German citizens.

With time on his hands, he began devising his system of exercises to train his body for health as well as strength. He began teaching other internees. As an orderly in the hospital, he jury-rigged hospital beds, springs and pulleys into equipment to enable physical therapy for the patients. He eventually transformed these improvised contraptions into highly sophisticated pieces of exercise equipment such as the Pilates Reformer and the Trapeze.

It's said none of the internees working with him died of the

Spanish flu in 1918.

In 1925 he migrated to New York City and opened up a studio to teach his system of "Contrology." Fortunately for us, he chose a location close to a dance studio. He nearly starved, until one of the dancers tried him out.

Soon he was famous throughout the New York City dancing community. His students included Martha Graham and George Balanchine. Some of them became well-known Pilates teachers after their retirement from dancing.

Although Pilates himself was supposedly influenced by Zen Buddhism (which has nothing to do with physical exercise) and the Greek ideals, practicing Pilates itself comes with a lot less philosophy than yoga and qigong.

He believed in the power of breath, but it's practiced as part of the physical movements.

Much Pilates is much more strength oriented than yoga and qigong. It's certainly not weight lifting or calisthenics, but well-rounded and developed strength, especially in your midsection core, is a goal.

Pilates has a lot of equipment you can buy, but none is necessary. Joseph himself always had new students practice on the mat before they were allowed to use any the equipment.

So to benefit from Pilates you don't need to spend any additional money for equipment. Just practice on the floor or use the equipment only while in a studio.

I recommend walking an hour a day, then fitting yoga, qigong or Pilates into your schedule three or four days a week if you can.

If you can't, don't. It's as simple as that.

However, if possible I'm sure any one of those three would help you lose weight, look better and feel healthier.

And now you have greater energy and strength, you're ready to earn some Bonus Exercise Points. You can't spend them, but you'll lose excess weight even faster.

Chapter Seventeen

Interval Training

This chapter has to come under the category of Not Mandatory—or, An Additional Assignment for Extra Credit.

Because, to be fair, it doesn't quite fall under the "relaxation" category of weight loss.

Oh, it'll help you lose weight and it'll help relax you—when it's over.

But it may not be what you think you signed up for when you invested in this book.

I told you I didn't want you to lift weights and spend long, boring hours jogging or doing any other alleged "cardio."

And I stand by that.

What I didn't tell you (until now) is you'll lose weight faster and improve your health by spending short periods of time on intense exercise.

When done correctly, it's not boring, because you don't have enough energy to feel bored.

Forget "Cardio," and Really Improve Your Heart Health

It's not the long, drawn our mile after dreary mile endurance running or jumping around—or anything else commonly called "cardio" by today's mainstream media.

No, I want you to spend intense quality time improving your heart and lung capacity. No more than twenty minutes a day.

You can even do it while watching TV, though if you do it right you'll lose track of the story.

It's called interval training, wind sprints, PACE and other names.

The basic idea is to push yourself to capacity, rest a little, then repeat. For no more than twenty minutes at a time.

And when you're in good condition, you can shorten it to twelve to fifteen minutes. It's only beginners who need to take twenty minutes.

The weight loss benefits of intense workouts don't come from the calories you burn in twenty minutes (it'll feel like you must be burning more calories than you really are).

1. You rev up your metabolism rate. This persists for twenty-four hours unless you eat a high glycemic load meal earlier. That is, you reduce the benefit of this exercise if you eat the sweet and starchy foods we already know you shouldn't be eating. Thus, you burn a higher than average number of calories throughout the rest of your day and even at night while you're sleeping.

2. You increase your supply of human growth hormone or HGH.

As you remember, HGH makes you younger in every way, including lowering your body's fat percentage.

For men, high intensity exercise increases testosterone. This hormone is also important for maintaining health and youth no matter what age you are—including lowering your Body Mass Index.

3. By strengthening your heart, lungs and circulatory system, high intensity exercise improves your body's ability to take in and use oxygen. The better you use oxygen, the more fat you burn.

Just in case the idea of sprinting makes you long for a slow distance run, there's a reason I'm not recommending such exercise.

Long Slow Distance is Not Weight Loss Friendly

Long duration exercise is stressful (duh!). And remember our old enemy cortisol the stress hormone? Exercise does increase your body's levels of cortisol. For the first twenty minutes or so, the benefits of exercise outweigh the levels of stress. That's why we squeeze as much exercise as we can into that twenty minute period, and then stop.

Because if you continue after that, you're dramatically increasing your levels of cortisol.

And to me, it just makes sense we're not supposedly to jog or run for many hours a day.

Did our cave ancestors live like that? I doubt it. I suspect men walked just as far as they had to go to find some game. Then they had to sprint like hell to run it down and kill it.

And sometimes they had to sprint like hell to keep something from eating them.

I've read stories of Native American hunters trailing a wounded deer for many miles. Cave men didn't have guns or even powerful arrows, so most of the time they probably either killed or missed entirely.

And even if they did sometimes trail a wounded animal for miles, that doesn't mean they did it every day.

Or that they ran the whole way instead of walking.

Women no doubt walked for many miles most days to gather food and water. And sometimes had to run like hell to keep from being killed or captured by an enemy group.

So I can readily believe our healthiest forms of exercise are walking combined with periodic but short, intense sprints.

But let's keep to the issue of weight loss...

When you run, jog, cycle, ski or swim for long distances, you burn calories from stored fat. Sounds good, right?

Wrong!

Remember, the number of calories you burn during exercise are relatively insignificant. What's important is what your body does after the exercise is over.

When you force your body to burn calories during a long endurance run, you're sending a signal to your body it needs a HIGHER reserve of calories. You body has evolved to protect you from starving to death.

During high intense exercise of no longer than twenty minutes, your body is burning carbohydrates stored in your muscle tissues—not stored fat.

Once you stop eating, your body goes into afterburn mode. Instead of wanting to replace stored fat, it wants to replace stored carbohydrates in your muscles. And it does so by burning stored fat for as long as twenty-four hours following the exercise.

Unless you eat something sweet or starchy.

After you exercise is not the time to reward yourself with a can of soda or candy bar.

OK, let's get started.

I have to say. If you didn't listen to me at the beginning of this book when I said to consult your doctor first—

DO IT NOW!

Don't start a new exercise program, especially an intense one, without being checked out.

Now that you have your doctor's OK, you have to remember. You have to begin where you are.

Choose An Exercise You Enjoy, One That's Easy to Start

You can select any activity you like. I enjoy running, but you can cycle, swim, ski, run up stairs, perform pushups, use an exercise machine designed to handle speed, or just do jumping jacks.

You can also vary them. Run this week and swim next week. Run today when the sun is shining, do pushups inside when it's raining.

First of all, spend several minutes warming up. This can be any light exercise that gets your blood flowing.

You're going to go in cycles.

Short, intense exercise.

Rest.

Short, intense exercise.

Rest.

And so on.

To begin with, each cycle should be around five minutes total, so you do four of them in the twenty minutes.

Then warm down with some more light exercise, especially walking.

And you're done for the day.

If you're so out of shape that walking around the block is the most intense activity you can manage, then walk around the block.

Then rest.

Then walk around the block again.

If running slowly is the most intense exercise you can handle, run slowly for about a minute, then walk for four.

If you're near a hill, going uphill is a great way to increase the intensity.

Gradually increase the effort you put into the intense phase. So even if you're running slowly on a level surface now, in a few months you're sprinting uphill.

Gradually increase the amount of time you spend on the intense phase. So this month you can sprint for twenty seconds. Next month you sprint for thirty seconds.

Gradually reduce the amount of time in the resting phase.

Push Yourself, but Not Over the Edge

Pay attention to your body. If you're huffing and puffing, that's good. That's the idea. That shows you're pushing your heart and lungs to increase their capacity. And you can expect your muscles to feel the discomfort of lactic acid build up.

However, if you feel any pain in your heart, muscles or joints that is sharp and sudden or just plain wrong—stop and get help immediately.

Running this way reduces your risk of injuries and joint damage, but it can still happen. Running with a torn muscle just worsens the injury, increasing recovery time.

As time goes by and you build your muscles and increase the capacity of your heart and lungs, you can also decrease your total time spent exercising. When you're sprinting longer than you're resting, you can reduce your total time from twenty to fifteen.

When you're in really good shape, you only need twelve minutes to stay that way.

Ideally, you'd spend that entire twelve minutes sprinting uphill. I don't know if anybody is at that level of fitness. I'm sure not.

Do this three times a week—and only every other day. Preferably not two days in a row, though sometimes I do that on weekends. But certainly not three days in a row. More is not better. Give your body time to recover and improve between sessions.

Walk for an hour the other four days of the week.

And four to six days a week, work in your yoga, qigong or Pilates. They have many health benefits not covered by either walking or interval training.

I know that sounds like a lot, and it does take time. But yet the "hard" part takes up only one hour per week. Walking is fun and relaxing. Don't make it hard.

And yoga/qigong/Pilates focus on breathing, gentle movement and postures. They keep your flexible.

I understand many weeks you won't have time for this full schedule—I don't either.

You'll get the most benefit from walking and gentle exercise, so work those in first. If you have thirty minutes to add interval training, all the better.

Chapter Eighteen

Additional Reduce Stress and Lose More Weight Tips

I've covered the main points by now, but while thinking about all the aspects of losing weight by relaxing, I came up with a few more tips.

Stay Out of Fast Food Drive-Thru Lanes

Don't you just hate to wait? I do.

And I hate it when I hear the car in front of me take ten minutes to give a simple order because they don't know what they want and their children are screaming.

I hate listening to three different rap songs because cars ahead of and behind me are blasting out an unchanging bass pounding (I refuse to call it a "rhythm" because there's nothing rhythmical about rap.) at two hundred decibels.

I hate deciding I want to leave, but I can't because there's a concrete barrier between me and the rest of the parking lot, and cars lined up behind me. I feel trapped and desperate.

I hate trying to give my order to a voice crackling so bad I can't understand what they're saying.

So you should just stay out of fast food drive-thru lanes, because I hate them so much.

But isn't it just too much trouble to park, get out and go inside?

Yes, it is—so don't.

If you're out driving anyway, just drive right by it.

Be A True Couch Potato

If you're at home on the couch, stay at home on the couch. Don't get up to fix yourself something to eat. If you're really hungry, just grab something easy such as an apple.

Staying on the couch is one of my easy-off weight loss tips.

Feel like going into the kitchen? No, that's too hard. Just stay on the couch. You want to be a couch potato, stay there. If snack food can't walk to you, you don't want it.

The Most Important Meal of All

Eat breakfast. All the experts say so. They can't give a scientific reason for it, but it seems to work. Almost all participants in the National Weight Control Registry eat breakfast every day.

Maybe it works because it forces you to get up earlier, which forces you to go to bed earlier at night, so you get more sleep, which we've already seen helps prevent weight gain.

Or maybe it works because you don't feel so justified in eating donuts, bagels and other morning junk foods during your morning break.

Weigh Yourself, but Not Too Often

You hear contradictory advice from the experts on this subject.

I believe the every-day-is-too-obsessive school makes sense. But if you never weigh yourself you never know how much progress you're making or whether you're going backward.

Besides, 75% of people in the National Weight Control Registry weigh themselves weekly.

Yet our weight does vary from day to day for reasons such as water retention that have nothing to do with how much of your body is fat.

Do weigh yourself at the same time of day, and the same day of the week, but only once per week. Preferably when you first get up in the morning just before your morning bath or shower, with all your clothes off.

Celebrate when it's low. When it's higher than the week before, acknowledge that, love yourself and resolve to follow this program more strictly.

The Only Diet Pills to Take Are Health Pills

You may have noticed I have not written anything yet about diet pills.

The reason's simple—they're too much trouble.

I recommend you take nothing except a high quality multi-vitamin/mineral and pharmaceutical grade fish oil, which is becoming more widely known as a source of the Omega 3 essential fats we need for good health.

I believe a good multivitamin/mineral can help you lose weight by giving your cells the nutrition they need, preventing them from making you feel deprived so you eat even when you're not hungry.

When I say "high quality," I do mean high quality. The cheap, hard tablets you buy at discount stores aren't worth the time or money. They don't dissolve in your body so you can't absorb and use whatever nutrition may actually be in them. You excrete them out into the toilet bowl.

So you must take find a brand of vitamins with high absorbability.

For my money, the best supplements in the world come from X-Tend Life in New Zealand. You can order through their website.

Many diet pills contain something that promises to absorb the fat in your diet so you can have the pleasure of eating the fat without the pain of finding it deposited to your waist.

What they don't tell you is that absorbed fat is taken out of your body through your next greasy smelly gross bowel movement. Be warned.

Also, remember your body doesn't store fat because you eat fat. That's simplistic, old-school weight loss thinking. Your body stores fat when you don't drink enough water, don't breath in enough oxygen, and your insulin levels are too high. That's why you need to avoid eating starchy and sugar foods, and continue to drink lots of water and take your deep breaths every day.

For sure stay away from the "fat burner" types of pills. They work by jacking up your metabolism. They're essentially legal speed. They're not as dangerous as meth, but too close for comfort.

Some ingredients make sense. Chromium directly affects your metabolism of sugar, so make sure your multivitamin/mineral contains some.

Some exotic ingredients promise to reduce your appetite or speed up your fat-burning metabolism. Maybe some of them work in a safe and healthy manner.

Maybe so, but I'm not convinced, so my advice is just to take the easy way out and don't bother.

Remember, thin people don't have time to research diet pills—so why should you?

Remember, you're a thin person who just happens to have a few extra pounds you're in the process of losing.

One final tip is to go back to the chapter on cortisol and refresh your memory on what reduces it.

We've covered direct relaxation and meditation.

But other things work too. They're not directly related to weight control, but they're important.

Laughing.

Listening to relaxing music.

Massages.

So, hang out with friends that make you happy, listen to music and have good times together.

Just don't pig out with them.

Afterword

Now You're on Your Own—You're Ready to Become on the Outside the Thin Person You Already Are on the Inside

We've come in a long way in just a few pages.

Here's a brief run down.

First and most importantly, we decided to take responsibility for our current and future relationship with food—and to lose the weight we want to lose.

We've come to understand that no diet is magic. We can lose weight by eating with common sense. Cut way down on sugar, starches, and fatty foods.

Eat lean meat, poultry, fish, dairy foods, fruits and vegetables—in moderation.

We've accepted we're human being who sometimes make mistakes. When we do, we learn from them and keep moving toward better health and fitness.

We've established the close relationship between carrying excess weight and stress, especially through the hormone cortisol.

We've started taking ten deep breaths three times a day.

Followed by complete relaxation...during which we visualize ourselves as thin people. We live through mental movies of ourselves enjoying life as thin people.

We learned how to anchor this state of relaxation and inner thinness by touching the tips of our forefingers and thumbs.

And we have transformed every former "eat now" signal in our lives into a trigger that makes us feel powerful, healthy, proud, energetic, happy and thin.

We're getting at least seven hours of sleep every night.

We deprive ourselves only of guilt, blame and self-criticism.

We drink lots of water through the day.

We walk at least one hour a day, five days a week.

We practice yoga, qigong or Pilates four to six days a week.

If possible, we practice interval training three days a week.

We understand we'll lose weight faster by eating plenty of calories at least one meal a week. However, eventually we may reach a plateau. It's a natural step in the process. We know to just keep going.

And finally, we've learned other ways to take life easy—to lose weight by just remaining on the couch and not lifting our hands to pick up more food.

That's a lot. Yet, what could be easier?

Breathing instead of counting calories, relaxing instead of going to meetings, meditating instead of writing a blog or journal, walking instead of running long distances, yoga instead of weight lifting, drinking lots of water...

If only our jobs and families were that easy, life would be too simple.

I believe I've fulfilled my promise to you—I've given you a complete system of losing weight through relaxation.

Now it's time for you to fulfill your promise to yourself.

Take responsibility for your weight loss and your life.

Do it now.

Weight Loss Resources

1. National Weight Control Registry

nwcr.ws/

This is an ongoing scientific study of people who have lost at least 30 pounds and kept it off for at least a year.

It's full of interesting information about what the people did both to lose their weight and to keep it off.

2. Eating Healthily

I can recommend only the Zone books by Dr. Barry Sears. Even though I criticize him for ignoring the mental/emotional dimension of weight loss, I believe his eating program is by far the healthiest way to lose weight and stay healthy your entire life.

And THE ZONE is still the best technical explanation for how the Zone eating plan works. (Not that everyone wants all the technicalities - but some of us do.)

3. Deep Breathing

JUMPSTART YOUR METABOLISM: How to Lose Weight by Changing the Way You Breathe by Pam Grout

4. Relaxation and Meditation

THE RELAXATION RESPONSE by Herbert Benson

CREATIVE VISUALIZATION by Shakti Gawain

THE SILVA MIND CONTROL METHOD by Jose Silva

5. Self Image Psychology

PSYCHO-CYBERNETICS by Maxwell Maltz

Combine what Dr. Maltz calls the Theater of the Mind with deep breathing, relaxation and alpha meditation and you can't help but change your life to get what you want.

There're a hundred meditation/alpha/self-hypnosis/self-image CDs you can buy to help you, with weight loss and every other problem and goal you can think of.

6. Water

YOUR BODY'S MANY CRIES FOR WATER by F. Batmanghelidj

WATER: FOR HEALTH, FOR HEALING, FOR LIFE: You're Not Sick, You're Thirsty! by F. Batmanghelidj

7. Yoga

YOGA AND HEALTH by Selvarajan Yesudian and Elisabeth Haich

or there're many other DVDs and books available.

8. Qigong and Pilates

There're many good books and DVDs available.

9. Interval Training

PACE by Dr. Al Sears